THE WHOLE BODY
CLEANSE

Authored By

Ombassa Sophera

Introduction 5

A Natural Healing Process 9

The Spiritual, Mental and Emotional Cleanse 13

Cleansing the Physical Body Systems 24

The Internal Baths for the Colon 26

External Detoxing for the Skin 43

The 6-part Physical Body Cleanse 48

#1 Colon Cleanse 48

#2 Liver and Gallbladder Cleanse 52

#3 Blood and Lymphatic Cleanse 56

#4 Kidney-Bladder-Adrenal Cleanse 61

#5 Cardiovascular Cleanse 65

#6 Lung Cleanse 68

Restoring the Systems 72

Anti-Inflammation Foods 73

Self-Preservation 74

"I am alive. I thrive. I am living well."

Introduction

It is time to stand for nature. To fully appreciate how it feeds, heals, clothes and shelters us. Full appreciation means taking special care of ourselves, the land, and others.

Since before the days of Imhotep, a master herbalist, foremost physician and scribe, humanity has maintained an ongoing search for methods of preserving and fortifying our health--finding cures and remedies for illness and disease, by re-sourcing this treasure house provided for us through our home, the Earth.

For uncounted millennia, these methods included the use of mixtures, tinctures, therapies and diets composed of primarily plant-life. Herbs and the development of herbalism became the miracle of sustaining a long and healthy life.
And, as mothers knew innately how to nurture the newborns into adulthood, health practitioners and healers – throughout history, also developed a keen eye and smell for those flowers, trees, shrubs, grasses and bushes that could be used to cleanse the blood, close up a wound, lower or raise body temperature, and eliminate inflammations and toxins from the body.

The Whole Body CLEANSE is presented and fashioned to open the way for you to create for yourself, a continued and steady, cleansing process. This type of cleansing process serves you by inoculating your whole body systems (spiritually, mentally, emotionally and physically) on a daily basis, instead of waiting for dis-ease to occur.

Within each of us, is the innate wisdom to maintain optimal health and vitality. The human body innately knows how to be a catalyst for its own healing. Our bodies are one magnificent healing machine, built for resiliency to continuously restore, regenerate and renew itself, in spite of ourselves. Just imagine the possibilities when we decide to assist this powerful and inevitable process, by deciding what is best for our own lives.

Our choices are plentiful for selecting the perfect wellness routine. Taking the opportunity to glance back, absorb and appreciate the origins of herbal medicine affords us our rightful place as our own healers.

Purposefully detoxing our spirit, mind and emotions, naturally roots out issues buried deep in the tissues, into the forefront--to now be healed. Taking time to observe your old reality and identify what thoughts and emotions no longer serve your life, will begin to open the space to crystallize new thought into a healthy existence.

Remember, the aches, pains and concerns of your body are really YOURS to take charge of. Every time we get our mental clutter (stress) out of the way-- through sleep, meditation or simply being in the zone of "fun", we allow our bodies to heal. This method of decluttering, playfulness, laughter or stillness, will always initiate the process of healing any issues we find ourselves facing.

When any healing formulas are used to address a bodily imbalance, the body naturally releases toxins stored over the span of a lifetime, out of its fatty tissue. These toxins, which often show up as symptoms, naturally come up for release, in reverse order of how they originally occurred in the body, i.e., the most recent issues leading the way in this toxin release process.

Appreciation for where we are right now on our healing journey, begins with planting just one new seed (thought) of whole healing in our fertile mind. The vitality birthed through appreciation of self, breeds an abundance of health, wealth and joy.

The healthy path to wholeness is the one where YOU decide that what you KNOW about yourself and what's really best for your well-being.

Initiate your healing process today, by being courageous enough to cease living life as you have known it be and simply decide to see another view of reality---and then shift into it.

Ombassa Sophera

August 2016

> "Great things are happening around me, to me and through me!"

A Natural Healing Process

There are simple steps to bring your body back into balance and alignment during or after an illness. This alignment comes with committed intention to heal your situation completely.

Creating a daily routine using healing modalities including; herbs, rest, meditation, relaxation exercises, herbal baths, therapy and eating balanced meals (best suited for your unique body), will assist tremendously in your healing process.

There is much information available for research today, to assist you in discerning what foods, herbs and activities, work best for your specific body type, i.e. information about alkalizing the body, eating right for your blood type, etc.

What I want to offer here is that we have at our disposal, tools and methods to really find out from our own bodies what it truly desires from anything. From what we will consume to where we take our bodies, body wisdom is one of our greatest treasures.

Take some time to research kinesiology or "muscle testing". It is something God-given that simply works every time. So, with all the choices of consumables available today, we can now decide to let our bodies be our guides. Then, victory is inevitable.

The combination of herbs and foods provided below in **bold**, are suggested to be the core food and herbs of each specific cleanse. Careful consideration is needed as no one body system is the same physiology, (even in the same ethnic groups). So when choosing from the food groups it is important to scrutinize the list carefully for optimal results.

Decide how thorough or quickly you want your cleanse to occur, by discerning the intensity and precision by which you will use the information in this book. The results can be as outstanding as you choose it to be, according to the care and discernment in which you use the information offered.

The Whole Body Cleanse assist you in:

- Enhancing the Immune System
- Releasing fears, inhibitions
- Increasing Energy Levels
- Reinforcing Positive Attitudes
- Eliminating Sugar and Junk Food Cravings
- Detoxifying, Rejuvenating, And Strengthening the WHOLE Body
- Releasing Excess Weight
- Boosting Libido
- Enhancing Circulation
- Amplifying Clarity & Optimism
- Improving Skin Tone and Complexion
- Balancing PH Levels in the Body
- Regulating Body Functions

"*I am choosing to have a great day!!*"

The Spiritual, Mental and Emotional Cleanse

This cleansing process is most important, as it is the cornerstone of ALL HEALING. It is a time where one decides to take matters of their health, back into their own hands through their own natural, God-given healing abilities.

With lots of PURE intention, a bit of spiritual guidance, utilization of our natural resources, and focused breathing and meditation, we will restore our bodies to optimal health and well-being.

The Spiritual Self

After providing over 23 years of spiritual healing, I would be remiss, not to first include simple steps to cleanse your Spiritual Self, which kicks off The Whole Body Cleanse.

Here are some very simple steps to spiritually cleanse:

Step 1

Find a space that you feel speaks to your peace of mind. It can be indoors or outdoors. Clear this space of anything disruptive or otherwise, that does not serve your forthcoming healing process.

Step 2

In this process, colors sometimes prove to be effective in both focusing your energy within, while drawing upon the healing energies of that color. It is proven that colors generate success in life if used properly.

In your quiet space now, allow your mind to get still. Feel around inside yourself to see what color comes for you to focus upon. When the color shows up, you may light a candle of that color. If no color comes up, simply use white.

Step 3

If you have some white sage, frankincense or incense to light along with your candle, this tends to assist to clearing and preparing your space for your cleanse.

Step 4

Here is where you begin Freedom Writing, where you write about everything in your life that has negatively affected your spiritual vitality, freedom and growth. Ask yourself now: What's been bringing me down lately? Where do I feel stuck and disempowered? What ideas, people, places and things, no longer serve my highest good?

Be honest and forthcoming as you write. This will feel extremely liberating. Writing it all out, feels just as great (if not better) as sitting with a therapist. Only here, you are sitting with your highest and greatest counsel, your Creator God, your Source. Safe, secure and fully loved, in its purest form-- unconditionally.

So BE FREE with yourself in this step.

Anything goes in the land of "I AM", I always say. Meaning, that anything you choose in your world to be right, is perfect, whole and complete as your truth in the moment where you are.

Hence, when you arrive at Step 6 you will begin your Restorative Statements with "I AM...."(whole, complete, loved, anything you are now choosing to be).

Remember, what we say and think today, become our children of tomorrow (what we experience as reality, based on those thoughts).

You may stay in this space of Freedom Writing as long as you need. Just to be sure you allow all to rise up to be forgiven, released or resolved about yourself and others, before moving into Step 5.

Step 5

In this step, you will rip up , all you have written in little pieces. Place it all in something safe to burn it. As you burn, connect with all the colors of your flame. Notice the outline of flame and how the colors change. This is transmutation at its best. Connect with this highest form of change in this moment.

Feel the peace. Take some natural breaths of release and relief. Now when you are ready, let's move on to our final step.

Step 6

Resolving to the great I AM. We are all baby creators and are given the power and dominion over our bodies. To NOT accept this gift and treasure, is to laugh in the face of the energy that created us and universes, our Creator.

Each time we say I AM, we reclaim our power. Now is the time where you can use these words of power for your highest good.

Begin writing your Restorative Statements of Power, these are your affirmative thoughts. Keep them flowing, as you continue to write, invoking more thoughts and feelings, that move you closer towards the center of yourself, who you really know yourself to be. Not who others proclaim you are. Who you KNOW yourself to be, your highest and best self.

As you finished this love session with your soul, you are enriched, enlivened and ready to embark upon any challenge life offers.

To keep on track daily, keep in mind the following:

- Be in FULL GRATITUDE for every experience, both you call good and not so good.

- Keep love in the forefront towards everyone no matter what they've done.

- Be sure your intentions come from a place of love for self and others.

- Attitudes are contagious so keep the mind distracted with things that bring you JOY.

- Remember that there is nothing to forgive, if you allow people AND yourself, to live your own destiny to the highest capacity possible.

Now is the best time to continue forward in the Whole Body Cleanse process, because you have now reclaimed dominion over your body through this spiritual process. You are more in touch now and will discern which items listed in the cleanse, will work best for cleansing your body, since everyone's constitution is different.

The Mental Self

Stress has a stronghold over most people's lives, causing debilitating illnesses and dis-ease. Most people feel stress simply because their beliefs are in conflict with the way they are actually living their lives. In this most important step of healing the WHOLE SELF, you have the opportunity to examine your beliefs, such as your values and life goals, to reveal the root cause of any undesirable results you are experiencing with your health and well-being.

How often do you find yourself holding your breath with the thought that something negative may happen in your life? Take a moment now to breathe in deeply this breath of life. Watch how your body naturally is gifted with a quick release of the tensions of the day. Do this every time you are dealing with stress of any kind or just when you are reminded to and it will powerfully change the course of your day.

A large percentage of the human beings on this planet are walking around depressed, confused and dissatisfied with their lives due to stressful situations they encounter on a daily basis.

Understanding the true causes of stress ultimately leads to reducing its impact on your life. Learning what to eat, think and how to act, will result in experiencing a healthier lifestyle. If you find yourself currently facing a health issue, you can explore what the potential thought processes you are holding that may be in connection with your distress.

Oftentimes, this connection is very subtle, difficult to see. There are healthy checkpoints you can use to reveal these connections to send you well on your way to optimal health and well-being.

Just answering these few healthy checkpoints will open you up to a state of clarity about your present thought processes.

- Considering your life purpose: How can I serve better?

- Examining your willingness: What level am I right now in terms of my availability to life? Am I showing up at my highest potential in this moment?

- Observing thoughts: Am I living my truth? What is my truth? What are three words that describe me and how I interact with others on a daily basis? Am I allowing past hurts, fears in relationships define who I am today?

- Viewing your behavior: Am I rested, well-nourished and hydrated?

- Assessing your efficiency: What is one act I can perform this day to move my endeavors forward? Am I willing to be thorough in all that I do?

- Self-Love: Am I demonstrating deliberate movement and enthusiasm in my life?

- Excellence: Am I commanding excellence my existing state of affairs?

Beginning to adopt a new attitude about life and the possibilities of successful living comes through realization that we all have the God-given ability to heal our situations. Daily meditation, affirmative thought and energy healing, strengthens our spiritual, mental, emotional and physical bodies. Communing with our Creator more frequently through prayer and meditation, liberates us to expand into our true birthright of abundance in health, wealth and joy.

Consuming foods that minimize the amount of time and energy your nervous system spends in catabolic mode, which tears down the body, will maximize the amount of time and energy it spends in anabolic mode, which nourishes, heals, and regenerates the body. Nerves are very important for the neurological functioning of the body. The nervous system is your body's decision-making and communication center. The central nervous system is made of the brain and the spinal cord and the peripheral nervous system is made of nerves. Together they control every part of your daily life, from breathing and blinking to helping you memorize facts for a test. Your nerves reach from your brain to your face, ears, eyes, nose, and spinal cord then to the rest of your body.

Stress, is a feeling of emotional or physical tension that can come from any experience or thought that makes you feel frustrated, angry or nervous. It is the body's reaction to a particular challenge or demand. Stress also can affect your appetite.

Short-term stress leads to the release of hormones (corticotrophin-releasing hormone and epinephrine) which energizes, while suppressing the appetite.

In contrast, long-term stress leads to excess release of another hormone (cortisol). Cortisol stimulates the appetite and the desire to overeat.

When stresses persist unchecked, the intake of foods high in fat and sugar is often increased. These foods are instantly satisfying simply because of their familiar taste, or the subconscious memories of comfort they bring from past times, of eating during upsetting moments.

The result is that areas in the brain that produce and process stress and the related emotions are now repressed. With such a dominant process resulting from eating these foods, even though it may be short term, it can become more challenging to plan and choose healthy eating practices while stress still persists. The consequence is often that instant gratification ingesting becomes a pattern leading to excess weight gain and/or ill-health.

More healthful eating of nutrient rich foods, higher in fiber, and healthy essential fats balanced with exercise is the long-term solution.

Whenever you are feeling stressed, B vitamins and related foods, which are especially important to keeping the nerves and brain cells healthy and happy-- are swiftly depleted. Using plants and foods that calm and relax the body will assist in mental clarity to see things not always visible within the muddle of life occurrences. With full intention and commitment, the following plants and foods will assist you to tune in to your body wisdom, to effect a higher state of healing.

The Best Foods for Nervous System:

Avocadoes, Fresh Green Leafy Vegetables, Bananas, Blueberries, Blackberries, Walnuts, Cruciferous Veggies, Sweet Potatoes, Brazil Nuts, Buckwheat, Sardines, Eggplant, Salmon, Herring, Almonds, Millet, Whole Grains, Oats, Dark Chocolate

Herbal Formula:

Lavender Flowers, Passionflower, Oatstraw, Peppermint Leaf, Rosemary Leaf, St John's Wort Flowers, Lemon Balm Leaf, Hops Flowers, Kava Kava Root, , Valerian Root, Skullcap Leaf Decaffeinated Green Tea Leaf, Mullein Flowers, Sage Leaf, Spearmint Leaf, Korean Ginseng Root

The Emotional Self

From the time we are born, our emotions are intricately involved with our digestive systems. If we observe how a baby feels as they are nursing: they feel secure, loved and safe. This becomes learned behavior so it is no wonder at all, that we often feel deprived when we are not eating, or when we decide to limit our food intake.

As you embark upon your cleanse, it is helpful to observe closely how you are feeling about it, paying special attention to any sense of loss or deprivation.

To balance these feelings, you may decide to support yourself in other ways that will comfort you. Activities such as journaling, doing artwork, dancing, taking a bath, going to see a movie, reading a good book, spending time with friends or getting a natural facial or massage will serve to give you the sense of security, love and safety you may feel is absent in your healing process.

The primary thing to remember when doing an emotional cleanse is to take care to watch what you are ingesting when you are upset or stressed out. Adhering to the foods in the Mental Self Cleanse section keep your stress levels down and steer you away from "emotional eating".

> "Life is loving me well and I deserve it!"
>
> "I willingly release all stagnating patterns."

Cleansing the Physical Body Systems

The next step for optimal health is cleansing the physical body systems. While most people just focus on the liver and digestive system when doing a cleanse, it only makes sense to involve ALL of the eliminatory organs. A natural detox of ALL major organs is essential to maintaining optimal health. You can take vitamins, herbs, and minerals daily and still not see an improvement your health situation. This is because your colon is filled with putrid fecal matter and your liver cannot purge toxins out of your blood and perform its daily functions.

Most of us, have experimented with different types of water or juice fasting, but very few of these include a full body, organ specific cleanse. Although general juice fasting definitely provides overall benefits, targeted cleansing and detoxing takes advantage of certain herbs, and alternative health protocols to greatly accelerate the process -- particularly in regards to specific body systems and/or organs.

For the entire process to work, you MUST ALWAYS do the colon cleanse before the liver detox, or you risk having major toxins push back into the blood stream.

In the following six part process you are provided foods and herbs that are known to support the particular system addressed. It is wise to ascertain and discern which foods you will use for your cleanse based on the severity of your bodily condition. There is NO ONE, BLANKET APPROACH. It is time for all of us to become our own reference point as it pertains to our own self. With this in mind, carefully choose (with the assistance of a professional if needed) which foods and herbs in each cleanse you will use for optimal results.

In each cleanse, foods, herbs and other methods are provided. Some foods and herbs offered, are more alkaline than others, which ultimately fuel powerful results if these foods become the spotlight of your cleanse.

Included within this cleansing process can be **internal baths for the colon**, (enemas) and **external tub and foot baths** (cleansing and detox) for the body.

The Internal Baths for the Colon

Think of your colon as the waste management location of your physical body. Every cell and tissue in your body and the liver (the major organ that detoxifies), all rely upon a well-operative colon so that your body can cleanse of excess waste and toxins.

The colon is the last segment (five feet long) of our extensive digestive tube. It is where the last of nutrients and water from the food we eat are absorbed into our circulation and where most of the waste products are eliminated. On the average, a person could have up to 10 pounds or more of non-eliminated waste sitting in their large intestine.

Unused food stuffs that are left over from digestion of what is eaten, is sent to the colon to be carefully expelled from the body. When everything is working in an efficient manner, the colon not only handles all that is unused, it also absorbs leftover nutrients (such as vitamins, minerals, water and electrolytes) from all foods digested, directing them back into the body for good use. Our colon decides what to get rid of and what is nutritiously important to redistribute into the body.

Besides eliminating leftover food that the body does not absorb—it actually filters waste from our blood stream into the digestive tube to be eliminated with the feces.

The colon also holds most of the intestinal flora, the trillions of "good" bacteria so important to our healthy functioning body. This bacteria helps with detoxifying, digesting and regulating the immune system, and well as many more roles.

The optimal situation for doing any colon cleanse, is when the colon fails to accomplish elimination of its content. While cleansing, the colon will sometimes eliminate extra mucus and oftentimes there is so much of it, that it gets stuck to the walls of the colon, blocking the elimination of what actually needs to be evacuated. At this time, it becomes so blocked that the mucus turns into a thick layer onto the walls of the tract. Often when an internal bath such as a coffee enema, is done in this situation, what comes out looks like a black tar, like a tire substance.

The physical body becomes toxic for various reasons:

- The liver is sluggish and blocked from toxins stemming from ingesting drugs, alcohol, chemicals, environmental substances and also, negative thoughts and emotions.
- Lack of necessary energy in the body for the colon to perform its task **sufficiently** if your adrenals and thyroid are not working properly. A stress-filled life and a lack of sleep reduce the capacity of these very important energy-producing organs.
- The colon is blocked, affecting your liver and kidney excretory functions.
- Peristaltic movement - the muscle contractions that push food through and out of your colon is inhibited because your stomach lacks adequate amount of hydrochloric acid which can be

caused by regularly taking digestive enzymes that have this important stomach acid (HCL).

Enemas

Enemas use pure water to hydrate the muscles of your colon, loosening up old, hardened fecal matter so that it can be safely eliminated from the body. An enema bathes your colon with pure water, along with whatever herbs, minerals or other healing agents you choose to use. It allows you to flush waste and cleanse your colon from the privacy of your own home. It is basically a way to hydrate and irrigate a section of your intestines by filling it with warm water and then flushing it out repeatedly, until elimination of waste in that session is satisfied. Simply put, an enema cleans up the colon and induces bowel movements, leaving you feeling cleaner, lighter, and healthier almost immediately. Even if you're feeling great, releasing extra toxins with an enema can make you feel better.

Reasons to Use Enemas:
- Colon Cleansing
- Liver Cleansing
- Fasting

I highly recommend enemas to people who are doing a cleansing program because, under these conditions the body often needs to expel greater amounts of this type of mucus fast, to eliminate constipation.

Two Types of Enemas: Cleansing or Retention

There are two types of enemas:
- The cleansing enema is retained for a short period of time until your natural peristaltic movement eliminates both the water and loosened fecal material. It is used to gently flush out the colon.
- The retention enema is held in the body for a longer period. Coffee enemas are retained for approximately 15 minutes or can also be left in and absorbed.

Cleansing Enema Types and Uses:

Most cleansing enemas are soothing and easy to use. An exception to this would be **Acidic/Astringent**✷ Astringent substances are used to shrink mucous membranes, causing a discharge. They are felt as 'drying'. The astringent substance is often, but not always acidic. They may also be antiseptic, and/or anti-inflammatory. If you have never done one of these before, I highly suggest using the lowest recommended amount of substance the first few times.

✷Apple Cider Vinegar Enema:

For detoxing & pH balance, also for use with viral conditions and clearing mucous from the body, nasal congestion or asthma. It releases toxins from the liver and has helped arthritis patients, people with high blood pressure, and skin conditions. Other ailments helped by consuming apple cider vinegar are high cholesterol, insomnia and fatigue, liver and kidney problems, candida and more.

Note, however, that candida will return in the next 24 - 48 hours, so this is not a permanent fix but rather provides temporarily relief from the symptoms. Be sure to take lots of probiotic foods (yogurt, kefir, sauerkraut, etc.) right after this enema to help restore proper microbe balance. You can also follow this enema with a probiotic enema or a probiotic implant.

✳Lemon Juice Enema:
Cleans colon, balances pH and detoxifies. If using for detox, alternate lemon juice enema with coffee enema on different days.

Warm Water Enema:
Cleansing the bowels

Aloe Vera Enema:
Good healing treatment for inflammation of the bowel.

Burdock Root or **Red Clover**: Eliminates calcium deposits and purifies blood.

Catnip Tea: Relieves cramping, constipation, congestion and fever.

Retention Enema Types and Uses:

Coffee: Stimulates liver and gallbladder to release toxins.

Minerals: Rebuilds energy of the adrenals and thyroid. Retains permanently.

Epsom Salt: The high amount of magnesium relaxes the muscles in the tract, increasing the amount of water that causes a thorough cleansing for those experiencing severe constipation.

Sea Salt (Saline) Recipe: Useful for softening old fecal matter because it can be held for a longer period of time.

Probiotic: Candidiasis and other yeast infections.

Red Raspberry Leaf: High in iron, particularly helpful for women.

Acidophilus Recipe: For those experiencing symptoms of IBS, constipation, hemorrhoids or other colon dis-ease.

Salts and Soda Recipe: Assists bodily conditions related to acidity, restoring acid-alkaline balance in the body.

Each enema requires a slightly different method. When a smaller amount of liquid is retained permanently, this is an implant (as used with the mineral enema). One cup of liquid with a probiotic, minerals, or something green with chlorophyll (like wheat grass) makes an excellent implant. They all will quickly have you on your way to a happier, healthier colon!

Recipes for Cleansing Enemas

Warm Water Enema

Ingredients:
  2 - 4 quarts warm, filtered water

Directions:
  Pour 2 quarts of warm water into enema bag, Allow to cool. Hang bag and insert tip (coconut oil is a good lubricant), allow fluid to flow into bowel, massaging abdomen to get all the fluid in.
Lie on floor/in bed on right side for 5 minutes, massaging abdomen; roll over to left side for another 5 minutes, continuing to massage abdomen. Then expel into toilet. Repeat with another 2 quarts of warm water, if desired.

Aloe Vera Recipe

Ingredients:
  1 cup pure Aloe Vera juice
  4 - 5 cups filtered water

Directions:
  Bring water to a simmer; allow to cool. Add aloe juice, then pour into enema bag. Hang bag in and insert enema tip (use coconut oil to lubricate it). Allow fluid to flow into bowel, massaging abdomen in counter-clockwise direction (up left side, across top, down right side, across bottom). Remove tip; lie in bed on right side for 5 minutes, massaging abdomen; roll over to left side for another 5

minutes, continuing to massage abdomen. Then expel into toilet.

Apple Cider Recipe

Ingredients:
    2 quarts filtered water,
    1/2 - 4 Tbsp apple cider vinegar.

Directions:
Pour 2 quarts of warm water into enema bag, Allow to cool, then add vinegar. Hang bag. Insert tip (coconut oil a good lubricant), and allow fluid to flow into bowel. Repeat, if desired. This enema may be difficult to retain more than 2 cups at a time.

Lemon Juice Recipe

Ingredients:
    2 quarts warm, filtered water,
    juice of 1 - 3 lemons

Directions:
Warm water, then cool. Juice 3 lemons, and stir into the slightly cooled water. Pour mixture through a mesh filter into enema bag; allow to cool. Hang an insert tip (coconut is a good lubricant). Allow fluid to flow into bowel, massaging abdomen to get all the fluid in. Hold for 3 - 4 minutes before expelling into toilet. You can lie on a bed or the floor and lightly massage abdomen if needed during the holding time.

Caution: If you've never done a lemon juice enema before, start with the juice of just one lemon, per 2 quarts of water as lemon juice is very astringent, and your body will want to get rid of it quickly, before getting much into your colon. Do a preliminary enema of 2 quarts warm water, to remove most stool first, before doing the lemon enema.

Herbal Enema Recipe:

Ingredients:
   2-4 Tbsp or 4 teabags of desired herb
   2 liters filtered water

Directions:
Add the herb to the water in a pot and bring the mixture to a boil. If it is the root or seeds, reduce the heat and simmer for 15 minutes, if not simply turn off pot and steep until cool to an appropriate temperature. Strain the solution and administer the same as instructed for previous recipe. Retain the solution 15- 45 minutes.

Recipes for Retention Enemas

Coffee Recipe

Ingredients:
1 liter warm, filtered water
3 tablespoons organic coffee

Directions:
In a saucepan, put organic coffee and add filtered water.

Boil coffee in water for 3 minutes, then reduce heat and simmer 15 minutes. Cool to desired temperature. When it is body temperature (you can test this by placing a clean finger into the coffee, it will be neither hot nor cold) strain into a clean glass jar and pour into enema bag.
Administer enema and retain for at least 15 minutes up to 40 minutes. Bring to the boil and let simmer for 15 minutes.

Notes:
Coffee enemas are the most powerful whole body enema detoxifiers. I recommend these for any disease that threatens well-being because unwanted invaders of the body system. For this reason I may speak a bit more on this one. Due to some amazing compounds within coffee that stimulate the liver to produce Glutathione S transferase, a chemical which is known to be the master detoxifier in our bodies, this enema binds the toxins and then releases them out of the body.

Reasons to use a Coffee Enema:
- To reduce levels of toxicity tremendously
- Cleans, heals, and improves peristalsis in colon
- Increases energy levels, improves mental clarity and mood.
- Helps with depression and sluggishness.
- Helps eliminate parasites and candida.
- Improves digestion, bile flow, eases bloating
- Detoxifies the liver and helps repair the liver
- Can help heal chronic health conditions (along with following a cleansing regime)

•   Helps ease detox reactions during periods of fasting or juice fasting, cleansing or healing.

Even if you're sensitive to caffeine, this won't affect you like drinking coffee will. (Decaf coffee will not provide the same benefit.) To ensure a thorough cleansing, administer another coffee enema within 6 hours to remove any bile released into small intestine not eliminated in the initial enema. Coffee administered by enema goes directly to liver, Because of this, be sure to only use organic coffee particularly ones developed specifically for enemas. Buy some premium ground ORGANIC coffee beans and keep them in the freezer until you need to use the coffee.
Do your coffee enemas as early as possible in the day to ensure no caffeine effects. After 6 weeks, cease coffee enemas for at least 3 months so that you will not deplete the body of minerals and vitamins it needs.

Epsom Salt Recipe

Ingredients:
2 liters warm filtered water
4 tablespoons Epsom salts

Directions:
Add Epsom salts to warm water, mix well until salts are dissolved. Administer and retain for as long as it is comfortable for you (see directions for administering below).

Notes:
Don't use if you are experiencing any:
- Nausea
- Vomiting
- Stomach pain

Never use more than one Epsom salt enema per day.

Salts and Soda Recipe

Ingredients:
2 liters warm filtered water
2 teaspoons sea salt (I prefer Himalayan)
1 tablespoon baking soda

Directions:
Mix until dissolved. Administer and retain for at least 10 minutes up to 30 minutes. If you are constipated, deliver only about a cup of solution at a time, until you have emptied your colon (the water runs out clear). For the first cup or so, don't try to hold it more than 5 minutes before voiding. If you are not constipated, lie on side and hold as long as possible,

10 - 15 minutes, massaging abdomen gently in large counter-clockwise circles. Then expel into toilet.

Note: You can do just the salt, without the soda, for a very soothing enema.
 You can also take a salt and soda bath, to relieve symptoms during a cleanse: Mix 1/2 pound salt and 1/2 pound baking soda. Dissolve in hot bath water. Get into the bath and relax.

Sea Salt (Saline) Recipe

Ingredients:
2 liters warm water
2 teaspoons sea salt (preferably Himalayan)

Directions:
Mix until dissolved, administer retain as long as possible up to 60 minutes (see directions for administering below).

Notes:
Unlike using plain water enemas, using salt water will not draw electrolytes from the body and does not draw water into the colon, because of this it is useful for softening old fecal matter because it can be held for a longer period of time.

Acidophilus Recipe

Ingredients:
2 liters warm, filtered water
2 teaspoons or 5 dry capsules acidophilus

Directions:
Stir together, pour in enema bag. Administer enema and retain minimum 10 minutes up to 30 minutes (see directions for administering below).

Notes:
Will give gentle cleansing while replenishing beneficial bacteria in the colon. This one is also good to follow other enemas if you are a frequent enema user.

Probiotic Retention Recipe (Implant)

Note: This enema is retained to reestablish probiotics in your upper colon. It should be done ONLY after a cleansing 2-quart enema, such as a salt & soda enema described above.

Following proportions, mix up only 2 cups. It's also a good idea to use a bifidus probiotic, as this is the most common beneficial bacteria in the colon.

Ingredients:
2 cups warm filtered water
1/2 Tbsp yogurt or kefir and/or 1 -2 capsules of bifidus probiotic

Directions:
Get a Davol tube to deliver liquid high in the colon. Best position for inserting this enema is on hands and knees, resting your head on your hands. Once delivered, roll onto your back for 5 - 10 minutes, massaging abdomen gently. Then roll onto left side before getting up. Hold as long as possible, at least

15 minutes, to give the bacteria a chance to take hold. Ideally, you won't expel it at all, except with your next bowel movement. If you have an urge to expel earlier, you may do so.

Enema Equipment

Purchase a quality enema kit to use for your enemas (if you buy a traveler's kit as it's easy to store and discreet for traveling). For the Probiotic Recipe implant you will need a Davol colon tube (you may purchase one at enemasupply.com).

Administering your Retention Enema

The first thing to know is that, if you are administering a retention enema, it would be ideal to do your enema after a bowel movement, so you can retain the liquid longer. If you are constipated, still the enema anyway, to get things moving along. Follow only directions for the desired enema stated above, if it has specific instructions. Otherwise you may administer your retention enema in the following manner.

Instructions:

Head to the bathroom with your bag and set up a space and something comfortable for you to lie down on. Hint: Be near a toilet and use an old towel as you sometimes may get slight leakage.
Now assemble your enema kit. It must have a tube and nozzle attached to the bucket or bag. Make sure it's at least 3 feet above you. (Hanging on a towel rail or shower rail is a good idea.)
There will an attachment near the nozzle that allows you to stop or start the flow of liquid once you have poured it into the bag. Ensure this is in the off position before pouring the liquid into the bag.
Once the liquid is in the bag hold tube and nozzle over sink or shower plug and turn it on and allow the liquid to run through the tube until there are no air bubbles. Stop the flow again once this is done. Get a pillow, soothing music or something to read and get as comfortable as possible.
Apply some coconut oil to the nozzle for easy insertion. Lie down on your towel on your right hand

side with your knees drawn up (You can also roll over to other side during the enema and do deep massaging to the colon area).

Insert the nozzle till it is about 1 inch inside the rectum. Turn on the flow of liquid slowly until the bag is emptied.

Now you can either remain lying on your side or lie on your back with your feet up above head level or feet resting against a wall above head level. You can even do some yogi moves, this helps get the liquid moving.

Relax and let things flow for time specified in the directions.

Try to retain the enema for allotted time period. You may feel some strong urges to go to the toilet, especially the first few times you try this. Breathe deeply and focus, holding on for as long as you can, sometimes this will help those sensations to pass. As you enemas more regularly you will be able to retain for longer.

When you are ready to release head to the toilet and let it go. You should feel a lot lighter now.

Enema Kit Care

To keep your enema kit in tip-top shape clean with a mild detergent and ensure everything is dry before packing away.

External Detoxing for the Skin

Using Clay for Detoxing

Types of Clay:

- Bentonite clay– bentonite clay usually forms from weathering of volcanic ash, most often in the presence of water. Bentonite clay has some antibacterial properties that help to combat acne and is a powerful detox agent.

- Green clay – green clay is loaded with iron and magnesium which gives it its green color. It acts fast to absorb oils and toxins, and is suitable for oily skin.

- White clay – also called kaolin. This is a very gentle clay, and is suitable for sensitive, dry and mature skin. It softens, exfoliates and purifies the skin. It has many benefits including antibacterial and detoxification properties. This type of clay can be used on a daily basis to help clean the skin and remove toxins and dirt from the pores and helps to regenerate cells in the skin.

- Fuller earth – this is a clay-like earthy material that absorbs bacteria and toxins. It is used as a body or face mask and has a slightly gritty texture that is great for exfoliating. It also has antiseptic properties.

Uses of Clay:

- Taking clay orally to detox your body:

  Bentonite clay is a powerful detox agent. It is naturally absorbent and gentle on the body's systems. It contains a certain mineral called montmorillonite, which is believed to be the primary component responsible for its health properties. It also contains magnesium and many other trace minerals that attract all sorts of toxins, including bacteria, heavy metals and pesticides. It enriches and balances the blood, absorbs radiation and neutralizes poisons in the intestinal tract.

  This clay is very versatile, and is used to treat a large number of physical conditions, such as bloating and constipation, food allergies and food poisoning, colitis, viral infections and parasites, helps to detoxify the liver, cleanse the colon, strengthen the immune system, alkalize the body and helps to improve the bacterial balance in the digestive tract.

  How to use bentonite – bentonite clay comes in a powder form. Mix 1 tsp of the clay powder into eight ounce glass of water and drink the mixture on an empty stomach and at least one hour before eating or taking other supplements or herbs. This is because you don't want the clay to interfere with the absorption of beneficial nutrients in your food.

- **Applying clay to skin**

  You can use clay externally during your cleanse, by applying a paste of clay and water. To make a

paste, add water to the clay until you get a paste
that holds together and doesn't fall apart. Leave it
on until it dries and then wash off.
Clay removes the dead layer of skin and draw
toxins from the skin. On a deeper level, clay wraps
given by a clinician, can relieve joint, rheumatic
and arthritis pain.

External Detox Bath (foot or tub)

Before, during and after your cleansing process, include this detox bath for peak cleansing results.

Ingredients:

> **2 cups Epsom Salt (or Sea Salt)** draws out toxins from your body while relieving aches and pains

> **1 1/4 cup Apple Cider Vinegar** soothes and softens dry, itchy skin while balancing the bodies and neutralizing the pH in the body.

> **1/2 cup Bentonite Clay** stimulates the lymphatic system and deeply cleanses your skin, the body's largest breathing organ

> **5-10 drops of any four the following Essential Oils**

Lemon, Rose, Geranium, Rosemary, Ylang Ylang Grapefruit, Tangerine, Orange, Juniper, Cypress, Rosemary, Mandarin, Lavender, Geranium, Palmarosa, Patchouli, Peppermint, Rose, Sandalwood, Fennel, Fir Balsam

Directions for Use:

Run your bath water as hot as you can comfortably take it. Add your bath components and agitate water to dissolve completely before stepping in. Soak for 20-40 minutes. I recommend a nice candle, doing some breathwork (deep breathing) and prayer, while you are enjoying your bath! Be sure to drink lots of water once you are done.

"*I flow with the ever present joy of life*"

The 6-part Physical Body Cleanse

#1 Colon Cleanse

Our digestive systems digest and absorb nutrients from foods. It also eliminates wastes by way of the the gastro-intestinal tract and the liver. It is great to give our entire alimentary canal an occasional break and boost, with a cleanse or fast.

There are different methods you can use to cleanse your colon-through foods, herbs, enemas and a more in-depth fashion: hydrotherapy (colonics). If you choose to cleanse using herbs and foods, due diligence is required in choosing those that work well with your body's constitution. Guidance is most often required in getting to know the best products to ingest.

Using plants and foods will help condition your colon and intestinal tract by mildly stimulating peristalsis, (due to its mucilaginous and bulking action effect). A clean colon and optimum functioning colon is a must for optimal health and wellbeing.

The Best Foods to Cleanse Your Colon:

Spinach, Kale, Broccoli, Turnip Root, Rutabaga Yogurt, Flax Seed, Citrus Fruits, Strawberries, Irish Moss, Watermelon, Honey Dew Melon, Apples, Cilantro, Cabbage, Beets, Brussels

Sprouts, Turnips, Cauliflower, Alfalfa, Wheatgrass, Chlorella, Barley Grass, Spirulina, Miso, Sauerkraut, Barley, Quinoa, Oats, Beans, Peas, Rice, Barley, Sweet Potatoes, Brown Rice, Barley, Carrots, Cantaloupe, Kefir

Herbal Formula:

Senna Leaves And Pods, Cascara Sagrada, Carbon (Activated Charcoal), Buckthorn, Black Walnut Hulls, Slippery Elm Bark, Marshmallow, Peppermint, Bentonite Clay, Cape Aloe, Goldenseal, Rhubarb, Irish Moss, Mandrake, Ginger, Poke Root, Psyllium Husk, Cayenne Pepper, Guar Gum

In addition to the Herbal Formula here are other essential things to consider for ultimate wellbeing for the Digestive System:

- Eat in peace and with intention to chew your food well. Do not to eat when you are nervous, rushed or stressed.

- Your goal whether you are cleansing or not needs to be at least one bowel movement every day.

- Add probiotics to the digestive system after cleanse by slowly introducing fruits (apples, grapes) and vegetables, such as live sauerkraut.

- Digestive bitters can also be very helpful to encourage the proper functioning of the GI tract.

- Bentonite clay has a negative ionic charge that allows it to bind with anything in the GI tract with a positive charge such as bacteria, viruses, and toxins. It is then removed from your body through the digestive system. Use only bentonite that specifies for internal use. Take one teaspoon (if you have the powdered clay) and mix it thoroughly in at least 8 ounces of water. This blend can be take 1-3 times a day with a half of lemon. Be sure to drink lots of water (at least half your body weight per day)!

- Psyllium seed is a natural bulking laxative that helps to improve bowel function and carry wastes out of the body via the GI tract. Mix 1 teaspoon psyllium in 8 ounces of water and drink 1-3 times a day. Psyllium needs to be used carefully as tends to block the system if not used with the correct herbs and liquids. Always drink this mixture quickly as it starts to thicken soon after it is mixed.

- An enema is the act of instilling liquids into the rectum. Use warm, purified water or herbal teas when making an enema. Doing a coffee enema brings tremendous healing and detoxing results for those more serious issues in the body. I highly suggest getting at least three colonics during your cleanse.

"My life reflects a pure existence."

#2 Liver and Gallbladder Cleanse

There is a very important reason that we focus on the liver when doing a cleanse. It's because it is one of the most important detoxifiers in the body. It helps "sort out" the blood and creates bile, a waste product that is crucial in the digestive process.

Using plants that consist of the highly efficient hepatic (liver-specific) herbs along with the foods below, will assist you to cleanse, strengthen, tone, rejuvenate, restore, maintain, and nourish this most important organ.

You cannot live optimally with a polluted liver- your body's first line of defense organ. The liver is greatly compromised with excess ingestion of chemical toxins from foodstuffs (i.e. meat, packaged foods and junk food), also consuming toxic drugs and unknown chemicals that we breathe or consume secondhand.

The Best Foods to Support Your Liver:

Apples, Flax Seeds, Lemons, Limes, Turmeric, Artichoke, Raw Vegetable Juice, Onions, Leafy Greens, Garlic, Grapefruit, Beets, Avocados, Brussels Sprouts, Cilantro, Parsley, Beet Greens, Dandelion, Asparagus, Broccoli Sweet Potato, Blackstrap Molasses, Bananas, Tomatoes, Spinach, Olive Oil, Quinoa, Millet, Chia Seeds, Buckwheat, Apple Cider Vinegar, Lentils,

Herbal Formula:

Milk Thistle Seeds, Dandelion Leaf and Root, Artichoke, Yellow Dock, Liverwort, Oregon Grape Root, Chlorella, Burdock Root, Sarsaparilla, Turmeric, Green Gentian Root, Fringetree, Peony Root, Goldenseal, Mandrake, Chicory, Agrimony, Yarrow, Wormwood, Hops, Artichoke, Barberry

In addition to the Herbal Formula here are other essential things that support ultimate wellbeing for the Liver and Gallbladder System:

- Digestive Bitters are herbs that taste bitter and stimulate the digestive system and liver. They act as a wonderful tonic, encouraging proper digestion and can be used daily. Approximately 15 minutes before each meal, place 10-15 drops of a tincture of digestive bitters on the tongue to enhance the digestive process. Hepatics are liver tonics and strengtheners. They can help stimulate liver function.

- If you are a person that tends to have digestive or liver issues, using a bentonite clay pack or *castor oil pack (see kidney section) daily over the liver during a cleanse can be helpful.

- *Liver Flush stimulates the liver function and helps the gall bladder flush.

*Liver Flush
- 1 cup fresh citrus juice (avoid grapefruit)
- 1 tbl extra virgin olive oil
- Dash of Ginger and Cayenne
- 1 clove garlic

Drink this formula first thing in the morning. One half hour later, drink 2 cups of Kidney Formula (see above). Wait another 1/2 hour and then eat your delicious, whole, organic foods that you have chosen for your cleanse (see above).

"I flow with the currency of gratitude.
My life force flows freely."

#3 Blood and Lymphatic Cleanse

The blood is a combination of plasma (watery liquid) and cells that float in it. It is a specialized bodily fluid that supplies essential substances and nutrients, such as sugar, oxygen, and hormones to our cells, and carries waste away from those cells, this waste is eventually flushed out of the body in urine, feces, sweat, and lungs (carbon dioxide). The lymphatic system sorts through the fluid from our cells and is an integral part of the immune system. We can think of it as our filter system on a cellular level.

Using plants and foods will help nourish, strengthen, tone, rebuild, maintain and purify the blood and lymphatic fluids of toxic waste and impurities. This formula will remove toxins and impurities from the blood and lymph.

The Best Foods for the Blood/Lymph:

Dark Leafy Greens, Broccoli Sprouts, Flaxseed, Basil, Blueberries, Cilantro, Cabbage, Apples, Beets, Strawberries, Lemons**, Turmeric, Basil, Garlic**

Coriander, Cilantro, Broccoli Sprouts, Broccoli, Parsley, Dandelion Greens, Avocado, Pineapple, Oranges, Papaya, Carrot

Herbal Formula:

Yellow Dock, Burdock Root, Dandelion, Red Clover, Sassafras, Chaparral, Neem, Cleavers, Goldenseal, Oregon Grape Root, Nettles,

Cayenne, Sarsaparilla, Cat's Claw, Pau D' Arco, Cerasee, Calendula, Mullein, Red Root, Chickweed, Red Root, Strawberry Leaf, Amla Fruit,

In addition to the Herbal Formula here are other essential things that support ultimate wellbeing for the Blood and Lymphatic System:

- Eat good quality fats and avoid margarine and fried foods.

- Drinks that are deep red, such as cranberry, beet, and pomegranate nourish the blood.

- Making a smoothie or drink daily, that includes a green food such as chorella (rids heavy metals), spirulina (reduces blood-fat levels), and barley grass, these are all great sources with alkaline properties that supports healthy pH balance, are rich sources of chlorophyll, a traditional blood cleanser and builder

- Irish Moss is packed with minerals and will prove valuable in nourishing the blood (muscle test your body for this and anything else you have question about to be sure it will be compatible for your body with all the recent talk of it containing carrageenan, which is said to produce inflammation).

- Omega 3 essential fatty acids are especially important for proper lymph function. Use a good quality fish oil that has been tested for heavy metals or fresh flax seed oil. Other oils that are highly beneficial include cold pressed olive oil and unrefined coconut oil.

- Lymphatic massage, which incorporates a light touch, will significantly help lymph circulation.

- Consider yoga, walking or swimming to move the lymph during cleanse.

- Dry brushing is excellent for encouraging lymphatic circulation. When dry brushing, use a soft natural bristle brush and always brush starting at the extremities and moving toward the heart. You can use essential oils in this process by first getting wet in the shower. Turn the shower off and add a few drops of essential oils listed below to your body brush. After brushing your entire body (but avoiding the face), wait for 20 seconds and then turn the shower back on and rinse well.
- Rebounding or jumping on a mini-trampoline can stimulate lymphatic drainage.

- Hot-Cold showers are an invigorating way to move the lymph. The last minute or so of your shower make it hotter than usual. Then the last 30 seconds turn the water to tepid. When you leave the shower you shouldn't be cold, but refreshed.

- Essential oils best to include for the lymph are: Cypress, Grapefruit, Orange, Sandalwood, Myrtle, Lemongrass, Tangerine, Rosemary and Cedar.

- *Make a lymph oil to use with your massage.

- If you tend towards swollen lymph nodes, try to get a lymphatic massage during your cleanse and incorporate dry brushing into your morning routine.

*Lymph Massage Oil -This oil can be used to massage in a small amount directly over swollen lymph glands or behind the ear and down the neck for ear infections. For a full body lymphatic massage, dilute the prepared oil below in 3 ounces of Almond and/or Jojoba oil before use.

Ingredients:
- 10 drops Lemon essential oil
- 10 drops Geranium essential oil
- 10 drops Rosemary essential oil
- 10 drops Eucalyptus Globulus essential oil

> "*Living is a sheer delight and I am happy with my life partners.*"

#4 Kidney-Bladder-Adrenal Cleanse

The urinary system includes two kidneys, two ureters, the bladder, two sphincter muscles, and the urethra. Your body takes nutrients from food and uses them to maintain all bodily functions including energy and self-repair. After your body has taken what it needs from the food, waste products are left behind in the blood and in the bowel. The urinary system works with the lungs, skin, and intestines—all of which also excrete wastes—to keep the chemicals and water in your body balanced. The kidneys help to maintain the body's pH balance. They eliminate wastes from the blood, keep electrolytes in equilibrium, and maintain water balance and blood volume.

The following plants and foods will help cleanse, nourish, strengthen, revitalize, restore, maintain, and tone the kidneys and bladder, ensuring optimal health and wellbeing of these important members of the urinary system.

The Best Foods for Urinary System:

Cranberries, Garlic, Blueberries, Blackberries, Red Radish, Celery, Cucumbers, Broccoli, Cabbage, Brussel Sprouts, Turnips Greens and Root, Kale, Rutabagas, Cauliflower, Dark Leafy Vegetables, Asparagus, Carrots, Mung Beans, Yogurt

Herbal Formula: Juniper Berries, Cornsilk, Uva Ursi, Buchu, Cranberry, Cleavers, Celery Seed, Parsley Leaf, Gravel Root, Nettles, , Goldenrod, Devil's Claw, Dandelion leaf, Burdock, Cubeb Berries, Couchgrass, Pipsissewa, Horsetail, Agrimony, Hydrangea

In addition to the Herbal Formula here are other essential things that support ultimate wellbeing for the Urinary System:

- Drink plenty of water, at least half your body weight of water in ounces every day.

- Avoid alcohol, sodas, caffeine.

- Avoid juices unless they are fresh and low on the glycemic index (get a glycemic chart). Mix all fresh juice with 50% water before drinking.

- Diuretic foods such as celery and cucumber help to flush the kidneys and eliminate wastes through the urine.

- Enjoy a shot of fresh juiced cranberries or drink 100% juice from store.

- Applying a bentonite clay pack or a *castor oil pack over kidneys will help bring blood to the area and draw out wastes.

*Castor Oil Pack:

Castor oil packs can be very healing for any organ. They encourage better circulation and lymphatic drainage, both essential in maintaining tissue (and therefore organ) health. They help to heal wounds, infections and stagnant conditions, as well as digestive and reproductive issues and inflammations.

- Use a clean unbleached and undyed cotton or wool cloth.
- Saturate the cloth with castor oil and place the cloth on desired area and cover it with a large enough piece of plastic.
- Place a heating pad or hot water bottle over bag and relax for at least an hour (longer if desired).
- Store cloth in a bag in the refrigerator between uses.
- Cloth needs to be washed or disposed of when the oil starts to smell rancid
- Castor oil packs can be done from 3 to 5 times a week.

"I live love completely"

#5 Cardiovascular Cleanse

The heart, which normally beats about 100,000 times every day, is the primary organ of the circulatory system and is responsible for pumping blood throughout the entire body. The cardiovascular system transports oxygen, nutrients, hormones, antibodies and waste.

Using plants and foods will help strengthen, tone, restore, maintain, and nourish the heart and vascular system in addition to enhancing and improving circulation in the body. This heart cleanse also contains specific herbs and nutrients shown in studies to help the heart maintain its functional and structural integrity It will remove toxins and impurities from the heart, arteries, and veins.

The Best Foods to Support Your Heart:

Chia Seeds, Cinnamon, Flaxseeds, Almonds , Asparagus , Broccoli, Dark Leafy Greens, Oats and Oat Bran, Turmeric, Spirulina, Decaffeinated Green Tea, Broccoli, Citrus Fruits, Watermelon, Apples, Pears, Bananas, Oranges, Sweet Potatoes, Carrots, Persimmons, Orange Juice, Cinnamon, Salmon , Pomegranate, Sunflower Oil, Safflower Oil, Canola Oil, Decaffeinated Black Tea, Red Wine, Brown Rice, Quinoa, Barley, Avocados, Walnuts, Lentils, Chickpeas, Soybeans , Salmon, Halibut, Mackerel, Olive Oil

Herbal Formula:

Hawthorn Berries, Ginger, Angelica, Blessed Thistle, Horse Chestnut, Shepherd's Purse Cayenne, Garlic, Sorrel, Irish Moss, Butcher's Broom, Gingko Biloba, Green Tea, Lily Of The Valley, Bugleweed, Prickly Ash, Motherwort, Mistletoe (European),

In addition to the Herbal Formula here are other essential things that support ultimate wellbeing for the Cardiovascular System:

- Stay away from dietary fats, saturated fats, refined sugars, carbohydrates and meats.

- Whole grains, especially oats and oat bran, are high in soluble fibers that bind to and flush cholesterol from the system. Eating whole grains can improve digestion due to the presence of high levels of fiber. Avoid wheat and barley if you're gluten intolerant.

- Fresh fatty fish is high in heart healing omega-3 fatty acids which are shown to help lower blood pressure and reduce the risk of heart attacks.

- Pectin is a natural fiber found primarily in citrus fruits, apples. Pectin binds to cholesterol and helps flush it from the blood, eating apples can lower cholesterol levels greatly.

"I only look for good in every life situation."

#6 Lung Cleanse

The respiratory system of the upper abdomen and chest includes the structures involved in the vital delivery of atmospheric air and the exchange of gases between the body and atmospheric air. Your lungs are organs in your chest that allow your body to take in oxygen from the air. They also help remove carbon dioxide (a waste gas that can be toxic) from your body. For your lungs to perform their best, these airways need to be open during inhalation and exhalation and free from inflammation or swelling and excess or abnormal amounts of mucus.

Using plants and foods will help strengthen, tone, rejuvenate, restore, maintain, and nourish the lungs and entire respiratory tract/system so you can experience your optimal birthright of clear breathing. This formula contains the best lung-specific herbs that will help to restore and maintain your lungs.

The Best Foods to Cleanse Your Lungs:

Flaxseeds, Spinach, Asparagus, Citrus Fruits Strawberries, Broccoli, Pineapples, Cantaloupe, Watermelon, Raspberries, Blackberries, Blueberries, Onions, Cabbage, Celery, Cucumbers, Horseradish, Cauliflower, Kale, Pomegranates, Turmeric, Red Bell Pepper, Pistachios , Cayenne Pepper, Apples, Celery,

Carrot, **Garlic**, **Ginger,** Tomato Juice, Salmon,
Nuts, Beets, Lentils, Kiwifruit, Mango, Pumpkin

Herbal Formula:

Mullein Leaf, **Lungwort**, **Irish Moss**, **Eucalyptus**,
Coltsfoot, **Hyssop Licorice Root**, **Marshmallow**,
Cayenne, **Chaparral**, **Osha Root**, **Horehound**,
Elecampane, **Slippery Elm Bark**, **Yerba Santa**,
Oregano, **Wild Cherry Bark**, **Pleurisy**, **Thyme**,
Cinnamon, **White Pine Bark**, **Peppermint**, Lemon
Balm, Blackberry Leaf, Goldenseal, Boneset, Lobelia,
Comfrey Leaf,Black Cumin Seed, Magnolia,
Schizandra, Plantain Leaf, Fenugreek

In addition to the Herbal Formula here are other
essential things that support ultimate wellbeing for
the Respiratory System:

- Pistachios are known to be great for the lungs.

- The anti-inflammatory and antioxidant qualities
  of omega-3 fatty acids, found in high supply in
  salmon, mackerel, nuts, and seeds, can help
  reduce the symptoms and protect the lungs.

- Blueberries are well known anti-cancer and
  anti-inflammatory snacks that can help protect
  your lungs and prevent a variety of common
  infections.

- Ginger has long been used to remove toxins from the respiratory tracts, it also has strong anti-inflammatory, anti-cancer benefits that keep the lungs healthy.

- The active organic compounds in kale help decrease oxidative stress in the cells and organs in the lungs.

- The enzyme that the flavonoids in garlic stimulate, increases the efficiency of the lungs to rid itself of toxins and carcinogens, proving garlic to be a flavorful and effective means of detoxifying and protecting the lungs.

- Though its identified as one of the hybrid foods, the antioxidant activity of carrots is awesome, and can be a powerful line of defense against lung issues.

- Guava has a huge amount of vitamin C per serving, it is a must if you're susceptible to lung infections.

- Flaxseed speeds up the lung healing process.

- Apples are particularly rich in antioxidants, and also a good deal of fiber.

- Hydration is key for overall lung efficiency.

"*I restore my POWER to the HIGHEST level of love.*"

Restoring the Systems

After cleansing the body systems, restoration is required for optimal health and well-being. Inflammation is at the heart of most diseases, including diabetes, heart disease, asthma, stroke, chronic periodontitis, rheumatoid arthritis, hepatitis, tuberculosis, chronic ulcers, thyroids, migraines, Crohn's disease cancer, obesity, which lends to it being a leading cause of illnesses in the USA. Here is when you make the necessary adjustments to the body with plants that restore balance. Most imbalances are connected to inflammation in the joints and tissues.

The Process

Nature has given us some wonderful plants that can be used in your diet to alleviate all autoimmune and chronic inflammatory disorders to restore the body to good health. What you ingest has a lot to do with what happens next. While herbs are very potent in their anti-inflammatory properties, there are powerful foods known for their anti-inflammatory properties Being sure to intake a wide variety of these foods on a frequent basis will go a long way toward preventing chronic illnesses. Using anti-inflammatory foods and plants will alleviate this issue, restoring the body into balance.

Anti-Inflammation Foods

Fruits: Avocados, Guavas, Strawberries, Mulberries, Raspberries, Blueberries Goji berries, Cherries, Cranberries, Apples, Oranges, Kiwifruit, Rhubarb, Lemon, Limes, Papaya, Pineapples

Vegetables: **Ginger**, **Sweet Potatoes**, Swiss Chard, Green Beans, Bell Peppers, Kale, Bok Choy, Olives, Fennel bulb, Spring Onions, Mushrooms, Leeks Kefir, Kimchee, Miso, Tempeh

Cold-Water Fish: Cod, Tuna, Herring, Trout, Alaskan Salmon, Striped Bass, Halibut, Whitefish, Sardines, Snapper Fish, Oysters

Oils: Avocado oil Olive oil.

Seeds and Nuts: Walnuts, Linseed, Hazelnuts, Sunflower Seeds, Almonds

Spices and Plants: Cloves, Cinnamon, Jamaican Allspice, Oregano, Marjoram, Sage, Thyme, Cayenne, Oregano, Parsley, Rosemary, Basil, Turmeric, Boswellia, cloves, Marjoram, Oregano, Cinnamon, Thyme, Sage, Basil Leaf, Bergamot Leaf, Devils Claw, St. John's Wort, Willow Bark, Turmeric, Chamomile Flowers, Red Clover Leaf, Echinacea Leaf, Ginger Root, Rosemary Leaf, Yarrow Leaf, Sorrel Blossoms, Sheep Sorrel Leaf, Alfalfa Leaf

Self-Preservation

This is the first rule of nature. Taking time to first appreciate the journey you have taken yourself through is paramount to preserving on the onward road to optimal health and well-being. With lots of work and PLAY, you will find it a natural order of things to always take FULL responsibility for your own thoughts, emotions and ways of being that creates the new blueprint for your ultimate health and well-being!

EnJOY your new health and wellness journey!!!

LIST OF HERBAL SUPPLIERS

Starwest Botanicals

www.starwest-botanicals.com

Herbco

www.herbco.com/Wholesale-Herbs

Atlantic Spice

www.atlanticspice.com

Traditional Medicinals

www.traditionalmedicinals.com

Frontier Coop

www.frontiercoop.com

Mountain Rose

www.mountainroseherbs.com

Taos Herb

www.taosherb.com

A Journey of Wellness

Since 1988, Ombassa Sophera has combined years of herbal study, a legacy of home remedies, and wellness coaching, to provide viable solutions to leading rich, holistic and enriching lives.

In 1993, she founded The Natural Healers Network, a health event series for health and wellness practitioners in Atlanta, GA, which included: organic cooking courses, reiki, iridology and a host of other alternative health modalities. In 1997, she began facilitating her signature workshop entitled, "Taking Responsibility for Your Health and Well-Being".

Ombassa is dedicated to assisting you to awaken to your ultimate potential, dreams and aspirations. Her work encompasses balancing WHOLE BODY SYSTEMS, guiding you towards ultimate health from the inside-out, while creating new and improved blueprints for living your passion and purpose.

Ombassa's sessions consist of physical, spiritual, mental or emotional attunement and introduction to the use of customized herbal blends to balance and align the physical system The sessions target any life issue- physical, mental, emotional or spiritual, addressing and restoring personal power outages experienced daily.

Ombassa's philosophy: "while stress consistently has a stronghold on people's lives–causing; debilitating illnesses, relationship breakups, unhappiness and depression, the key to healing isn't just ingesting an anecdote of any sort, more importantly, it is also mandatory to purge yourself the thoughts and emotions that make these imbalances possible".

The author of three books—Soul Journey to Truth, Inspire Yourself and ABC's of Nature's Best Herbal Recipes, two meditation CDs—SolJoy in Love and Soul Journey to Truth, Ombassa also provides custom herbal consultations through her blog and conducts workshops on herbal medicine, mindfulness and self-love across the USA and abroad.

Contact Ombassa:

http://ombassa.com

info@ombassa.com

www.ingramcontent.com/pod-product-compliance
Lightning Source LLC
Chambersburg PA
CBHW060207290526
45789CB00003B/1203